MEN USAGl

(TADALAFIL)

The Ultimate Resource for Defeating
ED, Addressing Premature Ejaculation,
Restoring Strength, and Amplifying
Libido

Michael Levi

Table of Contents

Chapter One
Introduction to Cialis (Tadalafil)

Cialis, likewise known by its nonexclusive name tadalafil, is a physician endorsed medicine broadly used to treat erectile brokenness (ED), a condition that influences a great many men around the world. Erectile brokenness is the powerlessness to accomplish or keep an erection adequate for good sexual execution, which can have significant physical, close to home, and mental effects on a man's personal satisfaction. Cialis has a place with a class of drugs called phosphodiesterase type 5 (PDE5) inhibitors, which likewise incorporates Viagra (sildenafil) and Levitra (vardenafil). These medications are explicitly intended to work on erectile capability by expanding blood stream to the penis, working with the capacity to get and support an erection during sexual feeling.

Cialis is exceptional among its friends because of its more drawn-out term of activity — as long as a day and a half — which deserves it the moniker "the end of the week pill." This lengthy span considers more prominent adaptability and suddenness, settling on it a famous decision for men who don't really want to time their drug around arranged sexual action. Interestingly, other ED medicines, similar to Viagra, regularly last around 4 to 6 hours, requiring more cautious timing.

Tadalafil, the dynamic fixing in Cialis, was created by the biotechnology organization ICOS and advertised by Eli Lilly and Company. It got FDA endorsement for erectile brokenness treatment in 2003, and from that point forward, it has become one of the main medicines for ED universally, close by Viagra. Notwithstanding its utilization for erectile brokenness, Cialis is additionally supported for the treatment of two different circumstances: harmless prostatic hyperplasia (BPH) and aspiratory blood vessel hypertension (PAH). The blend of ED and BPH medicines makes Cialis a flexible drug for men who experience the two circumstances, as it works on urinary side effects and erectile capability at the same time.

Pervasiveness and Effect of Erectile Dysfunction

Erectile brokenness is a typical issue, particularly as men age. It is assessed that 30 million men in the US alone experience the ill effects of some level of ED, with the commonness expanding with age. As indicated by research, around 40% of men experience ED by the age of 40, and that figure ascends to 70% by the age of 70. Nonetheless, ED isn't exclusively an issue for more established men. Factors like pressure, uneasiness, melancholy, heftiness, smoking, diabetes, and cardiovascular illness can add to erectile issues even in more youthful men.

The powerlessness to keep an erection can truly affect a man's confidence, certainty, and connections. Sexual brokenness frequently prompts pressure, humiliation, and can make distance in close connections, further worsening the profound cost of ED. Thusly, powerful medicines like Cialis can assume a basic part in reestablishing sexual capability as well as in further developing a man's general personal satisfaction and mental prosperity.

The Turn of events and Endorsement of Cialis

Cialis was created following the outcome of Viagra, which was the principal oral PDE5 inhibitor supported for ED. Perceiving the interest for elective ED medicines, particularly those offering more prominent adaptability, the drug organization ICOS teamed up with Eli Lilly to put up tadalafil for sale to the public. Clinical preliminaries exhibited tadalafil's viability in working on erectile capability, and it was found to have an essentially longer half-life than sildenafil, which prompted its lengthy span of activity.

In 2003, Cialis was endorsed by the FDA for the treatment of erectile brokenness. Over the long run, its purposes extended, and in 2011, Cialis was likewise endorsed for treating the side effects of harmless prostatic hyperplasia (BPH), a condition generally connected with maturing that makes urinary issues due the growth of the prostate organ. The capacity to treat both ED and BPH with one prescription settled on Cialis a significantly seriously engaging decision for men encountering the two circumstances.

What's more, a connected type of tadalafil was endorsed under the brand name Adcirca for the treatment of pneumonic blood vessel hypertension (PAH), a condition portrayed by hypertension in the conduits of the lungs. This features the flexibility of tadalafil as a prescription that can address various medical problems.

Chapter Two
How Cialis Functions

Cialis works by restraining the compound phosphodiesterase type 5 (PDE5), which is tracked down in different tissues all through the body, including the smooth muscle of the penis. Under ordinary conditions, sexual excitement prompts the arrival of nitric oxide (NO) in the penis. This triggers an expansion in degrees of cyclic guanosine monophosphate (cGMP), which makes the smooth muscles of the penis unwind, permitting blood to stream into the erectile tissue. This expanded blood stream brings about an erection.

PDE5 separates cGMP, and by hindering PDE5, Cialis forestalls this corruption, permitting cGMP levels to stay raised. This supports the smooth muscle unwinding fundamental for keeping an erection. Nonetheless, it's essential to take note of that Cialis, similar to all PDE5 inhibitors, possibly works when a man is physically invigorated. It doesn't cause unconstrained erections; sexual excitement is as yet expected for the drug to be powerful.

Cialis versus Other ED Prescriptions

Cialis is frequently contrasted with other PDE5 inhibitors, especially Viagra (sildenafil) and Levitra (vardenafil). While each of the three medications work likewise by restraining PDE5, there are key contrasts that impact a man's decision of medicine.

Term of activity: One of the main benefits of Cialis is its more drawn-out length. While Viagra and Levitra are compelling for around 4 to 6 hours, Cialis endures as long as a day and a half, providing men with a significantly longer open door for sexual action. This drawn-out term offers greater immediacy, diminishing the requirement for exact timing.

On-request versus everyday use: Cialis is accessible in two dosing structures — on-request dosing (generally in 10 mg or 20 mg dosages) and day to day dosing (2.5 mg or 5 mg). The day-to-day dosing choice permits men to keep up with reliable degrees of tadalafil in their framework, giving nonstop treatment to ED and more prominent adaptability for sexual action. This is particularly gainful for men who are physically dynamic on numerous occasions a week or the people who don't really want to design their prescription around sexual movement.

Aftereffects and bearableness: Cialis is by and large all around endured, with normal secondary effects including migraine, heartburn, muscle hurts, and nasal blockage. In any case, Cialis has a marginally lower chance of causing visual aggravations, which can be an issue with Viagra. Moreover, the muscle hurts and back torment at times connected with Cialis are not as normal with Viagra or Levitra.

Cialis for Different Circumstances

Notwithstanding its utilization in treating ED, Cialis is likewise supported for treating harmless prostatic hyperplasia (BPH). BPH is a typical condition in more seasoned men, described by an expanded prostate that prompts urinary challenges, for example, continuous pee, trouble beginning pee, and frail pee stream. Cialis helps by loosening up the smooth muscle in the prostate and bladder, which works on urinary side effects and furnishes alleviation for men with both BPH and ED.

Moreover, tadalafil (in an alternate plan) is utilized to treat pneumonic blood vessel hypertension (PAH). PAH is an uncommon however difficult condition where the courses in the lungs become limited, prompting hypertension in these vessels. By loosening up these corridors, tadalafil decreases the responsibility on the heart and further develops practice limit in patients with PAH.

Prevalence and Worldwide Use

Since its endorsement, Cialis has become one of the most generally recommended prescriptions for erectile brokenness, with a large number of men all over the planet profiting from its belongings. Its long length of activity and adaptability in dosing settle on it a famous decision, especially for men who need a more unconstrained way to deal with sexual action.

In 2018, after the patent for Cialis lapsed, conventional variants of tadalafil opened up, making the medicine more available and reasonable for men all around the world. The accessibility of generics has additionally set tadalafil's situation as a main treatment for ED.

Chapter Three
Erectile Dysfunction (ED)

Erectile Dysfunction (ED), regularly known as ineptitude, is characterized as the powerlessness to accomplish or keep an erection adequate for palatable sexual execution. While intermittent hardships with erections are ordinary, tenacious issues that impede sexual movement can prompt huge profound trouble, relationship issues, and diminished personal satisfaction. ED is a typical condition, especially in men beyond 40 years old, and its predominance increments with age. In any case, it's anything but an unavoidable piece of maturing, and viable medicines are accessible.

Erectile Dysfunction can have different causes, both physical and mental, and frequently includes a mix of the two. The condition is a vital mark of in general wellbeing, as it could be an indication of hidden clinical issues like cardiovascular sickness, diabetes, or hormonal uneven characters. Understanding the reasons for ED is fundamental for both avoidance and treatment, as addressing the main driver can frequently prompt superior sexual capability and generally prosperity.

How Erections Happen: The Physiology of Erectile Capability

To comprehend erectile brokenness, it is vital to comprehend how ordinary erections happen. An erection is the consequence of an intricate collaboration between the sensory system, veins, muscles, and chemicals. There are three key cycles engaged with accomplishing an erection:

Sexual excitement and nerve signals: When a man turns out to be physically stirred, either through physical or mental feeling, the cerebrum conveys messages through the nerves to the penis. This triggers the arrival of nitric oxide (NO) in the tissues of the penis.

Vasodilation and blood stream: Nitric oxide causes the veins in the corpus cavernosum (the elastic erectile tissue in the penis) to unwind and extend, permitting more blood to stream into the penis. As the veins widen, the expanded blood stream makes the penis grow and turn out to be firm, prompting an erection.

Supporting the erection: When the penis is engorged with blood, the veins that regularly permit blood to leave the penis become packed, catching the blood inside and keeping up with the erection. This cycle go on until sexual feeling stops or discharge happens, after which the blood streams out of the penis, and the erection dies down.

This series of occasions depends on solid vascular, brain, and hormonal frameworks. Any disturbance to these cycles, whether because of actual harm, ailments, or mental elements, can prompt erectile brokenness.

Reasons for Erectile Dysfunction

Erectile brokenness can result from an assortment of physical, mental, and way of life factors. Frequently, numerous contributing elements are available, making the finding and treatment of ED complex. The significant reasons for ED can be sorted as follows:

Actual Reasons for ED

Cardiovascular infection: ED is firmly connected to coronary illness and other cardiovascular circumstances, for example, hypertension (hypertension) and atherosclerosis (solidifying of the courses). These circumstances decrease blood stream to the penis, making it challenging to accomplish or keep an erection. As a matter of fact, ED is many times thought about an early advance notice indication of cardiovascular issues.

Diabetes: Men with diabetes are at a lot higher gamble of creating ED, as high glucose levels can harm veins and nerves that control erections. Diabetic neuropathy (nerve harm brought about by diabetes) and unfortunate dissemination add to erectile brokenness in diabetic men.

Hormonal awkward nature: Low levels of the male chemical testosterone, otherwise called hypogonadism, can cause ED. Testosterone assumes a key part in controlling sexual longing (moxie), and low levels might diminish a man's capacity to accomplish an erection. Other hormonal issues, like thyroid problems or over the top degrees of prolactin, can likewise influence erectile capability.

Neurological problems: Conditions that influence the sensory system, like various sclerosis (MS), Parkinson's sickness, stroke, or spinal rope wounds, can obstruct the nerve signals required for erections. Moreover, pelvic medical procedures (like prostate medical procedure) can harm the nerves answerable for erectile capability.

Meds: Numerous meds have ED as a secondary effect. Normal guilty parties incorporate antihypertensives (circulatory strain meds), antidepressants, antipsychotics, and certain drugs used to treat prostate malignant growth or harmless prostatic hyperplasia (BPH).

Substance misuse: The utilization of substances like liquor, tobacco, or unlawful medications can add to erectile brokenness. Smoking, specifically, harms vein and disables flow, while weighty liquor use can slow down the sensory system and hormonal equilibrium, prompting ED.

Mental Reasons for ED

Uneasiness and stress: Close to home and mental pressure can significantly affect sexual capability. Execution nervousness, specifically, is a typical reason for ED, where the strain to perform physically makes a pattern of uneasiness and inability to accomplish an erection. Summed up uneasiness about connections, work, or private matters can likewise add to ED.

Sorrow: Men who experience the ill effects of despondency frequently experience diminished moxie and erectile brokenness. The condition can make it challenging to take part in sexual action, and energizer prescriptions (particularly specific serotonin reuptake inhibitors, or SSRIs) can compound the issue.

Relationship issues: Issues inside a relationship, like absence of correspondence, unsettled clashes, or close to home distance, can influence a man's capacity to physically perform. ED may likewise demolish relationship issues, making a pessimistic pattern of sexual disappointment and profound strain.

Chapter Four
Way of life Elements and Erectile Dysfunction

Corpulence: Being overweight or hefty is related with a higher gamble of erectile brokenness. Abundance weight can prompt cardiovascular illness, diabetes, and hormonal awkward nature, all of which add to ED. Also, men who are large frequently have lower testosterone levels, further weakening sexual capability.

Actual latency: An inactive way of life can deteriorate dissemination and cardiovascular wellbeing, improving the probability of ED. Customary activity is gainful for further developing blood stream, decreasing pressure, and keeping a sound weight, all of which backing better erectile capability.

Diet: An eating routine high in immersed fats, sugar, and handled food sources can prompt circumstances like heftiness, diabetes, and atherosclerosis, all of which disable erectile capability. On the other hand, an eating regimen wealthy in natural products, vegetables, entire grains, and solid fats can assist with further developing blood stream and hormonal equilibrium.

Rest problems: Unfortunate rest designs, rest apnea, and ongoing sleep deprivation have been connected to erectile brokenness. Rest issues can disturb testosterone creation and lead to expanded feelings of anxiety, the two of which adversely influence sexual capability.

The Mental Effect of Erectile Dysfunction

The impacts of ED frequently reach out past the actual side effects. Men with ED every now and again experience mental pain, including sensations of disgrace, culpability, low confidence, and shame. This can prompt evasion of sexual circumstances and make strain in close connections. The close to home cost of erectile brokenness can be basically as critical as the actual difficulties, with numerous men expecting that they are at this point not fit for fulfilling their accomplices or feeling less "masculine."

ED can likewise add to relationship issues. Accomplices might feel confounded or dismissed, expecting that the issue is connected with an absence of want instead of an ailment. This misconception can prompt correspondence breakdowns and a reduction in by and large closeness. Couples really must talk about these issues transparently and look for clinical or mental directing if important.

Predominance of Erectile Dysfunction

Erectile Dysfunction is more normal than numerous men understand. It is assessed that roughly 30 million men in the US alone experience ED somewhat. Universally, concentrates on show that half of men beyond 50 years old experience some type of erectile trouble, and the commonness increments with age.

In any case, ED isn't simply a condition influencing more established men. Research proposes that roughly 20-30% of men under 40 experience some type of ED, frequently because of mental elements like pressure and nervousness, or way of life factors like smoking or poor actual wellness. The worldwide commonness of ED keeps on rising, driven by expanded paces of corpulence, diabetes, and cardiovascular illness.

Finding of Erectile Dysfunction

To analyze erectile brokenness, specialists normally start by leading a thorough clinical history, including conversations of side effects, way of life factors, and sexual wellbeing. Actual assessments may likewise be performed to distinguish any fundamental medical problems. Now and again, lab tests, for example, chemical levels, glucose tests, or cholesterol tests, are requested to evaluate potential ailments adding to ED.

In situations where mental variables are thought, specialists might allude men to a therapist or guide for assessment and treatment of uneasiness, gloom, or relationship issues. This can be vital for men whose ED comes from mental causes.

Treatment Choices for Erectile Dysfunction

There are numerous successful medicines for ED, going from way of life changes to meds and careful choices. These include:

Oral Drugs: PDE5 inhibitors like Viagra (sildenafil), Cialis (tadalafil), and Levitra (vardenafil) are ordinarily recommended. These meds assist with expanding blood stream to the penis, permitting men to accomplish and keep an erection.

Way of life Changes: Taking on a better way of life, for example, stopping smoking, getting thinner, practicing routinely, and eating a heart-sound eating routine, can work on erectile capability.

Psychotherapy: For men with mental reasons for ED, advising or mental social treatment (CBT) can assist with tending to tension, gloom, and relationship issues.

Chemical Substitution Treatment (HRT): For men with low

testosterone levels, testosterone treatment might be suggested.

Penile Inserts and Medical procedure: For extreme instances of ED that don't answer medicine, careful choices like penile inserts or vascular medical procedure might be thought of.

Vacuum Erection Gadgets (VEDs): These mechanical gadgets assist with bringing blood into the penis to make an erection and are much of the time utilized in mix with different medicines.

14560154R00024